MW01136694

by Sara McGinnis

This book was created by a writer, not a doctor, and is not intended as a substitute for the medical advice of physicians. The reader should regularly consult a physician in matters relating to his/her health and particularly with respect to any symptoms that may require diagnosis or medical attention.

Table of Contents:

"Courage is to tell the story of who you are with your whole heart.."

- Dr. Brené Brown

Introduction

It starts with a dull vibration in the body. A sensation in the arms that is not quite an itch but urges you to move and react all the same. Unbidden it buzzes through your limbs before dragging you down with an undeniable force, sapping your body of all energy. Everything feels wrong is all that you know, and in frustration you can't help but lash out, to do something, anything to change this feeling.

You wonder where the person you recognize as yourself has gone to, but no matter how hard you try and force her to reappear the waste of a human being you've become overnight refuses to let her return. A better person would find a way to keep this from happening again and again, you're sure of it, but every month you're dragged down so low, unable to stop it. This inability to do better, to be stronger, thereby serves as proof of how weak you truly are. A failure. Case closed.

Angry at yourself, and angry at the world, the unjustness and unfairness of it all consuming your thoughts, the rage begins to build. It's not an energetic rage though, but rather is a lethargic soaking that drenches your body in frustration causing you not to go completely wild, but to lash out instead at those you love most.

You start to wonder if you're losing your mind, and can't help but consider your family would be better off without you here with them.

This is life with PMDD, and it can be hell.

PMDD, which is the abbreviation for premenstrual dysphoric disorder, is a severe form of premenstrual syndrome which affects 3 to 8% of women. It's more than PMS. It's a debilitating, life-interrupting phase that occurs every month, complicating lives and harming relationships.

Over the past couple of months I've been talking to women on message boards and in Facebook groups about their stories, which are my story too. Welcome.

One — Life with PMDD

One week ago I took my bike down to the park and rode around the hilly, challenging five mile loop. My heart raced in time with the speed of my wheels and my body was energized by the cold wind in the air. Then I hopped off my bike and ran three miles through the wooded trails. I frickin' love running. I love the woods. I love being outside.

Two days ago a friend and I drove up into the mountains and hiked for five hours, first to an amazing waterfall, and then, because that wasn't enough, we climbed to the very top of the damn mountain. It was arguably the toughest hike I've ever been on, and I loved it.

This is who I think I am. An outdoorsy, adventurous, hard-working, responsible person who has a zest for life and can't wait to see what will happen next. I've got plans and get high just daydreaming about the sheer amount of possibilities out there.

But the next morning I woke up feeling wrong all over. The sky was still dark, but not as dark as my mood. Determined to make the best of it and have a productive day I threw on my slippers and made a giant, steaming cup of coffee. As I heard my kids awake I reminded myself to soften. "It is a normal day for them," I thought. "Be kind. Be patient. Be loving."

It worked, at first, as I typed away at the post I was writing for work while they clanked dishes about and got ready for school. I thought I could make it through to when the bus came to take them away, but then the rambunctiousness started. The big boy got the little boy riled up just for sport, and his choice of retaliation on what had turned into a bright and glorious morning was the helicopter bathrobe. Whipping his black garment of fleece around his head he laughed while making obnoxious sounds that translated to, "I'm gonna to get you!" Brother chased brother as squeals and laughter intermingled and overrode my request they calm down.

Some part of me could see they were having a great time, but when that bathrobe hit my giant cup of coffee, sending it off my nightstand and into the wall, splattering everywhere, I lost it. They froze as I shouted, "Argh! That was my goddamn coffee you hit!"

I am not normally a yeller.

No one moved, which infuriated me more. I jumped up from the bed, stomped into the kitchen and grabbed a towel as one child turned to hide in the bathroom under the pretense of brushing his teeth and the other scurried to his bedroom.

"Sorry?! Couldn't you at least say sorry? Offer to help?!"

The boy looking back at me from the center of his room choked out a sobbing, pathetic, "Sor - sniff - sorry!" I wiped up the coffee barely holding back the urge to yell and yell and yell some more. I felt small and terrible, completely defeated but yet somehow still itching for a fight.

I apologized on the way to the bus stop, and for the hundredth time silently gave thanks kids forgive and forget way faster than grownups do. That doesn't make it okay, of course, and in fact almost makes it worse. "One of these days they're not going to let it go so easily," I told myself. "What if all they remember of you when they're grown is this?"

Despite the terrible start to what ought to have been a lovely day I vowed to pull my shit together, but even the three-block walk home from the bus stop was taxing. The legs that could run miles and climb mountains days ago found the small trek exhausting. Safe inside the house I slumped into the couch, and rather than get to work as my schedule demanded, I cried. At first a trickle, and then full-on sobs as the self-loathing thoughts whirled into high gear:

> "What kind of a mom yells at their kids like that?"

> "Your life is so good, and yet all you can do is cry like a mopey asshole."

> "Fail. Fail. Fail. How much longer do you think you can hide what a failure you are from everyone else?"

One of the worst parts about having your own thoughts attacking you is they have the insider advantage. The voices that appear to pound you into the floor don't have to guess what your sore subjects are. They know each and every tiny speck of guilt and insecurity you harbor and have no qualms about using them against you. It fucking hurts.

I don't want to live like this, with the thoughts and the mood swings, but for now it doesn't seem as though I have much of a choice. There are some things I have found that have helped over the last couple of years though, and I'd like to share them with others who might be struggling.

A look at what Wikipedia has to say about the symptoms of PMDD:

> Premenstrual dysphoric disorder (PMDD) is a severe form of premenstrual syndrome (PMS). Like PMS, premenstrual dysphoric disorder follows a predictable, cyclic pattern. Symptoms begin in the late luteal phase of the menstrual cycle (after ovulation) and end shortly after menstruation begins. On average, the symptoms last six days, with the most intense symptoms happening in the two days before through the day of the start of menstrual blood flow.
>
> Emotional symptoms are generally present, and in PMDD, mood symptoms are dominant. Substantial disruption to personal relationships is typical for women with PMDD. Anxiety, anger, and depression may also occur. The main symptoms, which can be disabling, include:
>
> Feelings of sadness or despair, or even thoughts of suicide
>
> Feelings of tension or anxiety

Panic attacks

Mood swings or frequent crying

Lasting irritability or anger that affects other people

Lack of interest in daily activities and relationships

Trouble thinking or focusing

Tiredness or low energy

Food cravings or binge eating

Trouble sleeping

Feeling out of control

Physical symptoms, such as bloating, breast tenderness, headaches, and joint or muscle pain

The symptoms occur during the week before menstruation, and go away once it starts.

Want to hear something a little bit funny? It's no laughing matter, of course, but the page goes on to say: "A diagnosis of PMDD requires the presence of at least five of these symptoms."

Five? Ha! I've got that beat by a country mile, with all of the points listed being fitting descriptors of my monthly fallouts aside from panic attacks, trouble sleeping and physical symptoms. However, I feel strongly it's not the mere presence of some (or all) of these symptoms that makes PMDD so difficult, it's the intensity with which they appear.

I recently asked a group of online friends to describe their PMDD-induced emotions and experiences in just 5 words. It's a challenge to cut down so much to just the bare essentials, but here's a revealing look at what they shared:

>Crippling tears, failed yet again.

>Depression, anxiety, no real reason.

>Uncontrollable rage, hate being touched.

>Unworthy. My family deserves better.

>I just want to die!!!

>Unending tears - hell on earth.

>Doom darkness death destruction pain.

>Pain anger depression and worthlessness.

>This isn't who I am.

>Disgust, rage, guilt, anxious, annoyed.

>Depressed, useless, hopeless, distressed, possessed.

I hate who I become.

Another friend of mine recently told me her story, and agreed to let me publish it here. Reading her words I'm both amazed by how much they sound like me and saddened. As great as it is not to be alone I don't actually want anyone else to feel this bad either. She wrote:

> PMDD is ruining my life. Ruining my kids' lives.
>
> I hate everyone when it's here. It's a monster. It's evil. It's a curse. It's out of control. I rage. So much anger. I'm hostile. Reactive. Emotional. A mess. I swear.
>
> I have road rage. I can't think. I get paranoid. Noises are louder. Lights brighter. Smells stronger. My boobs hurt and tingle so bad it gets me down. I make poor decisions. I can't bare to be touched. My skin itches and crawls. My blood tingles. Restless legs. Mind races. I have nightmares. I'm fat. I crave carbohydrates & binge eat.
>
> I'm a vile creature.
>
> I ostracize myself. I want to hide in bed. I can't be bothered to bathe, to do my hair or makeup look nice. Brush my teeth.
>
> I feel low. Tearful. I'm in a dark hole. Brain fog. Can't concentrate. Can't communicate with

anyone. I feel lost. I wish I could end it all...It's exhausting. COMPLETELY exhausting. Debilitating.

Then.....one day....I wake up and boom....I feel happy (after I've had my period). I'm nice. I laugh. I have a spring in my step. I'm calm. I can think clearly. I look good. Smell good. I'm patient, kind. All is good.

But the realization of the damage I've caused while having PMDD is there, I hate myself.

I read on a PMDD forum that a lady felt like gouging her ovaries out with a spoon. I get that. If I could, I'd take it all out tomorrow.

How would you describe your experience with PMDD? Join the conversation by tweeting to me @Sara_McGinnis with the hashtag #talkPMDD.

Two — Meeting the Beast

"Sadness" and "despair" were not always words I would have chosen to describe my hormonal days, but the past few years they creep on like inevitable clockwork. Sure, there was "shocked" and "disbelief" when I first discovered what having PMS and my period was like at the age of 13 (Every month? Women really live like this?!), but early mood swings and cramps were nothing compared to the PMDD I would come to know a decade later.

Back in the days when I had PMS, like so many women do, I was irritable leading up to my period. I felt frustrated with things that weren't going my way, and every once in a long while snapped at someone I loved. One of the only fights my longtime BFF and I have ever had took place when I, for reasons that remain diluted by time, insisted on singing along with her favorite song like an asshole. I changed the lyrics, mocked the style and took my always off-key crooning to new heights all in an effort to -- I don't even know. To be a jerk, because I felt jerk-ish, I guess.

It was stupid and dumb (sorry BFF!), but seriously, that was the extent of my PMS. Every once in a while I was kind of a mild jackass for no reason, but life moved on pretty easily.

Between the time I was an early middle-school girl up to my first suspicions I was dealing with Premenstrual

Dysphoric Disorder I grew up, graduated, graduated again, got married and birthed two babies in 10 years time. It was a whirlwind, to say the least.

In the interim I'd dabbled in birth control, as is par for the course for those participating in sexual activities. I first hesitantly tried the pill, then switch to Depo and though that was unquestionably effective I put on over 20 pounds in a hurry. From there I went back to the pill, and two years after marrying at age 21 I quit all of it. We were open to starting a family and I was sick of taking birth control, and so we switched to condoms-only protection knowing we were rolling the dice a bit. Lucky for us, they worked until we decided to really try for a baby.

"I read that for most people it takes six months to a year to get pregnant," I informed my young, new husband as we drove home for Christmas break between his final semesters of college.

"So it will take a while?" he asked in reply.

"I guess," I answered, figuring I had no better gauge than the average to go by.

We had a very happy holiday season that year and two weeks after toasting to the new year I barfed. Not the I've-gone-and-drunk-myself-under barf of my previous years as a college student, but the early morning upchuck that sends your thoughts whirling and feet in motion towards the nearest store with a pregnancy test. Sure enough, the sex had worked.

Our first baby boy arrived roughly nine months later, and while I won't go as far as to say I was in bliss in my postpartum state, I was fine. My hormones were in check, I didn't feel as though I had PPD (postpartum depression) and between pregnancy and breastfeeding I didn't have a monthly cycle for nearly two years. It was amazing.

Unbeknownst to me at the time, I was pregnant with number two at our firstborn son's first birthday. Nine months and a few hee-hee-hee-hoos later I was the mom of two, and under the doctor's advice had a Mirena IUD implanted. I then embarked on a love/hate affair with my IUD, enjoying that I rarely had periods but ever so slowly I started to feel like I was losing my ever-loving mind.

There were headaches and low energy peppered with moodiness and anger, but I was also raising two children under the age of two! How was one to tell the root of any one frustration from another? And so I stuck with Mirena for years, growing increasingly tired of the way I was feeling but ultimately blaming myself for not doing enough to make my own life better.

"Maybe if you weren't so fat you'd feel better," the thoughts would hiss. "You're the one too lazy to actually do anything about it."

I did try, in spurts at least, to better myself. Like the time when I spent a seemingly gargantuan portion of the few dollars we had on a double stroller and started going for walks. That didn't last long though, and the workout intensity at the gym I later joined was just as sporadic. I could not, for the life of me, string together anything with consistency beyond two weeks.

Finally I had enough, and made an appointment to have the Mirena removed. We went back to condoms-only birth control, and then eventually my husband had a vasectomy.

After having my IUD taken out there seemed to be a brief roller-coaster ride of hormone ups and downs, followed by what, in hindsight, was a honeymoon phase. The headaches dissipated greatly, and at times I felt like my old self, catching hints of energy and enthusiasm for life. I felt like I was close to returning to how life as I had known it all along had been, and aside from some PMS here and there had no complaints.

But then, ever so slowly, my newly returned grasp on consistency and stability began to shake. In the early months what I believe was PMS being taken over by PMDD I acutely noted how 'off' I felt and how intensely I felt to change or fix the mood taking over. Seemingly out of the blue I would feel miserable, and was convinced doom was around the corner. Looking to relieve the mess of feelings and anxiety I felt building up inside of me a week or so before my period I turned to the tried-and-true, socially-approved, go-to release for women: wine.

I sipped, slurped and guzzled away from the feelings I could find no other way to relieve, and in the process of doing so ended up rottenly hungover. The relief I felt in the evening while three drinks in was long gone by the next morning, and in its place was not only a headache, sour stomach and exhaustion, but the beginnings of self-loathing.

But the funny thing about PMDD and the potent mixture of emotions surrounding it is that nearly as soon as my period started I felt real relief. I became absolutely convinced that I was through the worst of it, that I was back to being the me I knew so well, and that I would not fall so low ever again. It was like some sort of magical amnesia swept over me, told me that episode was just a fluke, and convinced me I'd be good to go from there on out. No need to worry even a moment more.

I don't suppose I need to tell you that's not how it works. Despite feeling just fine for a couple of weeks after my period, I'd inevitably fall into that dark space yet again.

For me, PMDD began as a tinge of rage complemented by feelings of failure and peppered with anxiety. Some months it was just a hint something was off, but other times it left me crumpled on the floor and left me unable to carry on with life.

I imagine, if pressed for a recipe sure to pull the rug out from under me, it would look a little something like this…

Ingredients:

Mix thoroughly:
¼ cup rage
⅔ cup failure
dash of anxiety

Blend in:

½ cup insecurity
2 packed cups lethargy
1 t. forgetfulness

In a separate bowl, fold together:
3 heaping scoops of shame
¼ cup impatience
4 t. insomnia
and 47 lbs of carbohydrates.

Layer in equal parts and sprinkle with 2 T.
general demons. Bake at 425 degrees until fuck
me.

While every month was a struggle there have been two particular days I remember being the very worst, in which I cried nearly nonstop. I shut myself in the bedroom and didn't come out until the next morning, alternating between sleeping and watching life happen without me. I sobbed when my husband played in the front yard with our two boys, and claimed I was sick when my in-laws stopped by to visit. I was deeply depressed and exhausted, but also angry at missing out on my life. I wanted to go out and join them, but the quivering rage in my veins left me not trusting myself to interact with anyone.

I wish I could remember where I first heard about PMDD, but alas I can't. However, I do recall it was probably close to two years from when I first heard of it until I typed those four letters into a search engine and broke down in tears reading the list of symptoms that described me all too well.

Here's a look at what some friends in an online support group I'm a part of had to say about how and when they first heard about PMDD. (All names have been changed to protect privacy.)

Elizabeth: I first heard of it two years ago when I was diagnosed. I had symptoms for probably a good 10+ years prior to being diagnosed properly. First it was major depression, then major depression with anxiety, then finally PMDD and Bipolar. But I'm not bipolar. It is only during those two weeks that I had a problem.

Carolyn: I first heard about it in 2008 or 2009, but suspect I've had it for much longer. My mother used to always time my periods by my moods when I was a teenager, and after the birth of my first child in 2006 it became much worse.

Lisa: I was diagnosed 6 months ago. After seeing 3 professionals that didn't know about PMDD and it seemed I had major depression. I couldn't understand why it happens before my period. I started looking for connections on the net. Then I came across PMDD. I found a clinic in Israel that deal with PMDD and didn't tell the doctor about my self-diagnosis. She and another specialist eventually came to the same conclusion. I've been suffering from it for 20 years. And the blame about not managing to control my mood before my period is starting to go away.

Ruby: I found it with Google during a bad PMDD week. I had symptoms since teen years that have got more severe after each of my three pregnancies.

Jessica: I heard about it about. 4 years ago, I think, but I have had it since I started my period (12 years old). I remember when I was a teen I would apologize to my friends at the start of the day saying that I was PMSing and not to take to heart anything I said because I would be snapping at them for nothing. My senses would be in overdrive and…I would get into these really down moods. I think it got worse after kids, though. After I had my son in 2003 my periods became really irregular and my symptoms skyrocketed. My symptoms would just build and build until I started my period.

Melanie: I only heard about it 3 years ago when I was at wits end with my moods. My doctor told me about it. I've had it since I was a teenager.

Three — But Why?

Why? seems an inevitable question. Why must this keep happening to us? Frustratingly, there isn't much of an answer.

Wikipedia states under causes: A demonstrable hormonal imbalance in women with PMDD has not been identified. It is hypothesized that normal ovarian function produces biochemical events in the nervous system that cause the premenstrual symptoms in women who have a predisposition to the disorder.

Mayo Clinic: The cause of PMDD isn't clear. Underlying depression and anxiety are common in both PMS and PMDD, so it's possible that the hormonal changes that trigger a menstrual period worsen the symptoms of mood disorders.

American Family Physician: Currently, there is no consensus on the cause of PMDD. Biologic, psychologic, environmental and social factors all seem to play a part. Genetic factors are also pertinent: 70 percent of women whose mothers have been affected by PMS have PMS themselves, compared with 37 percent of women whose mothers have not been affected.

NAPMDD (National Association for Premenstrual Dysphoric Disorder) goes on to explain how a woman's monthly cycle affects her by sharing:

The hormone progesterone is an essential part of the menstrual cycle, especially when it comes to reproduction. The rise in progesterone after ovulation is essential for maintaining a healthy pregnancy. When an ovulated egg is left unfertilized, progesterone falls and bleeding begins. This rise and fall post ovulation is called the Luteal Phase and typically when PMDD symptoms occur. In women without PMDD, progesterone has a near calming effect. Recent studies show that women with PMDD have an increased sensitivity to this particular hormone and experience increased activity in the emotional center of the brain. Much like some people drink alcohol and become happy while others become angry and violent.

They go on to explain "PMDD is a cyclical, hormone-based depressive disorder with symptoms arising during the luteal phase of the menstrual cycle and lasting until the onset of menstrual flow. It affects an estimated 2-8% of women of reproductive age. While PMDD is directly connected to a woman's menstrual cycle, it is not a hormone disorder."

I don't know about you, but it being a "hormone-based depressive disorder" but not a "hormone disorder" seems confusing as hell. I asked Amanda LaFleur, who is the founder of NAPMDD, what that means. Here's what she told me:

"I know it can be confusing and we are currently working on crafting a concise way to explain this disorder.

What is meant by PMDD is being a hormone-based depressive disorder but not a hormone disorder is that most women with PMDD have normal hormones. It is the way the mood center of our brains react to the natural rise and fall of hormones throughout our monthly ovulation cycle.

A hormone disorder would be someone who is, say, low in progesterone or too much estrogen. In this case the woman does not have PMDD but rather a 'hormone disorder.'

Having said this, a woman with PMDD can also have a hormone disorder but PMDD is not in itself caused by 'out of whack' hormones."

Hormone-based depressive disorders are going to include PMDD, pre and postpartum depression, perimenopausal depression and depression during menopause."

That's a little clearer, right? As NAPMDD works to clarify and explain they'll be updating their web site. I encourage you to check there, as well as follow them on Facebook for updates.

Nonetheless, their list of things that can help point to hormonally-based depression rings awfully true to me:

A history of mild or severe PMS as a teenager

Relief of depressive symptoms during pregnancy

Postpartum depression, with new-onset or newly recurring depressive symptoms

Recurrence of premenstrual depression following resumption of menstruation after delivery

Worsening of premenstrual depression with age, blending into the menopausal transition and becoming less cyclical thereafter

Coexistence of cyclical somatic symptoms, such as menstrual migraine, bloating, or breast pain which are not associated with bipolar disorder

Runs of 5 to 20 relatively stable mood state days per month

Recurrent episodes of depression, often severe and related to menstrual periods, but without episodes of mania

For me, the mild PMS as a teen, no symptoms during pregnancy, worse trouble with age, and amount of stable days all fit.

It was another few months after the self-diagnosis before I finally made an appointment with my OB/GYN. We had just moved to a new city and I had yet to set up a doctor through my provider. I'm not real good about going to the doctor on a regular basis, but from what I gather the woman in the white coat I met the day of my appointment was spectacularly bad at bedside manner.

Without thinking I had scheduled my appointment to coincide with the crux of my symptoms. In some ways this was a smart move because it meant I would be feeling the absolute worst, the peak of my symptoms, and would not be able to hide behind the forgetfulness that comes so easily as soon as my period starts. In reality though, it turned out to mean I was hot, crying mess in her office. When she asked if anything in particular brought me in that day the tears flow before I could even get a single word out.

"I'm ha-having a hard time," I blubbered out. "It's just that every month I'm falling apart. I can't stop crying and I'm angry — I'm not usually an angry person — and it's just so hard to understand what's going on."

I went on to explain to her that I had googled PMDD, read about the symptoms, and felt like that described what I had going on. Now I don't know if I'm just really good at self-diagnosing, or if I had thrown this OB/GYN off of her game, but after passing me the tissues to remedy this snot running out of my nose in a rather unladylike fashion she grabbed her prescription pad and said to me, "Is there a particular type of drug you'd like to try?" Just like that, with a few simple sentences, the pharmacy door was unlocked. It's not like I wanted to go through a long interview about all of my miseries with a perfect stranger, but I couldn't believe this was what being diagnosed was like.

"Maybe Prozac?" I asked. "Whatever you think is best?" Was I really the one that was supposed to be making the call here?!

Here's what NAPMDD has to say about the steps for a diagnosis:

> Whether you start with your Primary Care Physician or Mental Health Provider, your medical team should be working together to get you the correct diagnosis and treatment for your disorder.
>
> While there are no blood tests that can diagnose PMDD, a Comprehensive Female Panel blood test will rule out any underlying disorders that may be causing your symptoms. To get an accurate assessment, you will need to provide a detailed history of your symptoms including frequency and severity.

They explain the process further by sharing there are two routes to take.

Medical professional:

- Doctor visit: Visit your Primary Care Physician (PCP), General Practitioner (GP), or Gynecologist (OB). When finding a doctor to work with, don't hesitate to inquire about their background and knowledge of premenstrual disorders including PMDD.
- Blood test: Request a Comprehensive Female Panel to determine hormone levels and rule out

any other underlying disorders or conditions. Hormone testing should be done twice: once before ovulation and once after ovulation as hormone levels will naturally fluctuate during the cycle.
- Track Symptoms: Use a PMDD Symptom Tracker to track your symptoms from Day 1 of your menstrual cycle. A period of 2 months is best to determine if symptoms are tied to your cycle. A minimum of 1 month may be enough to determine a connection.
- Interpret Results:
    - Discuss medication options
    - Referral to Mental Health Professional
    - Diet and Nutrition and Exercise, referral to nutritionist
    - CAM: Complementary Alternative Medications/Treatments

Mental Health Professional:

- Doctor Visit: Make an appointment with your Therapist, Psychologist, Psychiatrist, or Counselor. When finding a doctor or therapist to work with, don't hesitate to inquire about their background and knowledge of premenstrual disorders including PMDD.
- Initial Assessment: Talk with your therapist about how you have been feeling and how long you have been experiencing symptoms. Be prepared to discuss your medical and mental history and answer questions as truthfully and accurately as you possibly can.

- Track Symptoms: Use a PMDD Symptom Tracker to track your symptoms from Day 1 of your menstrual cycle. A period of 2 months is best to determine if symptoms are tied to your cycle. A minimum of 1 month may be enough to determine a connection.
- Interpret Results:
    - Referral to PCP for blood tests
    - Discuss medication options and/or referral to Psychiatrist
    - Diet and Nutrition and Exercise, referral to nutritionist

CAM: Complementary Alternative Medications/Treatments

Four — Tiny Pills and Other Treatments

I went home after my awkward OB/GYN appointment with a small bottle filled with even smaller pills and two sets of directions. I could either take the pills only during half of the month, starting two weeks before my period and ending as soon as it did, or I could take them every day. Seeing as how I have no interest in taking pills on a regular basis I went for option one, with fingers crossed those tiny pharmaceutical bits could somehow grab me by the shoulders, lift me up, and keep me from falling off the cliff into the depths of PMDD.

In the second of only two blog posts I've written about PMDD thus far, I recalled of my experience with fluoxetine (which is also known as Prozac, Sarafem, Ladose and Fontex, etc.):

Two weeks from then, about the time my merry egg was estimated to be parting from my Fallopian tube, I popped the first pill — and fell asleep. I simply could not stay awake. I tried for a solid week to take those bad boys in hopes they'd boost me up over the hormone fallout, but slept nearly the entire time.

I suppose you could argue sleeping was better than raging on my loved ones, but it's hardly a reasonable way to get through life.

For the next few months I dabbled in trying to take the pills at night, before bed, as well as just on the days I felt particularly off. It was better, but they still left me exhausted.

Then, I did nothing. Life happened and we had to move again. I ran out of the pills and felt no desire to repeat my awkward office encounter, so I trudged on through a few more cycles. It was rough, and the month I outright told my family "I quit" and shut the door to my room for an entire day signified I needed to try again.

Shuffling to a new physician and scheduling my appointment during an 'up' time seemed to work out great, except that on the very-frowny face to crazy-happy face scale of questions I had to answer about my 'down' time the reality was bleak. Even on the "I sometimes think I can't go on like this any longer" question I had to mark the super sad face, but I clarified to my doctor that for me that didn't mean suicide — it meant me showing up that very moment in his office. For others, however, suicidal ideation is a monthly occurrence.

He was a great doctor, and prescribed sertraline (Zoloft). It also sucked.

I wanted so badly for it to be a magic pill, but it wasn't. I was willing to put up with some of the symptoms I experienced (mild fatigue, stomach cramping, cessation of sexual function) if everything else would be good, but then I couldn't sleep. I discovered that perhaps the only thing worse than exhaustion is insomnia.

And so I quit those, too.

I could have (should have?) gone back to the doctor and explained my frustrations, because I do know finding the

*right pill is a long process, but somewhere along the way
I began to realize I don't want to be on pills at all.
Antidepressants, birth control, or anything, if I can help it.
I don't like the side effects I feel, and am wary of those
that might not even be noticeable.*

I haven't been on pills at all in the year since writing that
post. I do, however, firmly believe that any person out
there who feels they are need of help ought to seek it
and, if need be, swallow what they're given with no
shame whatsoever. Do you. Whatever works. I doubt it's
worth much, but you have my blessing.

Seeing as how I'm not a medical person (please do
recall the opening statement in which I proclaimed
myself a writer and not a doctor, and that all medical
care decisions you make should be discussed with your
own physician) here's a look at what the experts have to
say about what is available to help those dealing with
PMDD.

Treatment options, according to NAPMDD, include
antidepressants, birth control pills, homeopathic
treatments, chemical menopause and
hysterectomy/oopherectomy. Below is further
information on each:

Antidepressants/SSRIs:

Several members of the selective serotonin
reuptake inhibitor (SSRI) class of medications
are effective in the treatment of PMDD. These
medications work by regulating the levels of the
neurotransmitter serotonin in the brain. SSRIs
that have shown to be effective in the treatment

of PMDD include: fluoxetine (Prozac, Sarafem), sertraline (Zoloft), paroxetine (Paxil) and citalopram (Celexa).

Up to 75% of women report relief of symptoms when treated with SSRI medications. Side effects can occur in up to 15% of women and include nausea, anxiety, and headache. SSRI medications to treat PMDD may be prescribed to be taken continuously or only during the 14-day luteal phase (second half) of the menstrual cycle. Other types of antidepressants (tricyclic antidepressants and monoamine oxidase inhibitors) and lithium (Lithobid) have not been shown to be effective in the treatment of PMDD. Finding the right dosage is key to the effectiveness of SSRIs. Many women with PMDD find a low dose to be more beneficial.

Oral Contraceptives (Birth Control Pills)

Medications that interfere with ovulation and the production of ovarian hormones have also been used to treat PMDD. Oral contraceptive pills (OCPs, birth control pills) can be prescribed to suppress ovulation and regulate the menstrual cycle. Certain combination birth control pills can offer some relief for PMDD symptoms.

Caution should be taken when considering OCP as many women with PMDD are sensitive to the hormone progesterone. All OCPs contain progesterone and may make symptoms worse. In randomized controlled trials, the only combination pills that have shown improvement in PMDD symptoms are pills that consisted of a combination of ethynyl estradiol and drospirenone (like Yaz, Ocella, and Beyaz). These pills have been shown to offer relief from both physical and psychological PMDD symptoms with improvement in health-related quality of life. For women who choose the Pill for contraception, Yaz is the only birth control FDA-approved to treat PMDD.

Homeopathic Treatments

In a controlled trial chasteberry extract (agnus castus fruit) was effective in decreasing the symptoms of PMDD. Several dietary supplements including calcium, vitamin B6, and vitamin E, have also been shown in limited studies to reduce PMDD symptoms.

Acupuncture has shown to have positive effects for physical pain and emotional symptoms including dysphoria and anxiety.

Chemical Menopause (GnRH Agonists)

Gonadotropin-releasing hormone analogs (GnRH analogs or GnRH agonists) have also been used to treat PMDD. These drugs suppress estrogen production by the ovaries by inhibiting the secretion of regulatory hormones from the pituitary gland. As a result, menstrual periods stop, mimicking menopause. Nasal and injection forms of GnRH agonists are available. Examples of GnRH agonists include: leuprolide (Lupron), nafarelin (Synarel) and goserelin (Zoladex).

The side effects of GnRH agonist drugs are a result of the lack of estrogen, and include hot flashes, vaginal dryness, irregular vaginal bleeding, mood changes, fatigue, and loss of bone density (osteoporosis). Adding back small amounts of estrogen and progesterone can help avoid or minimize many of the annoying side effects due to estrogen deficiency and help preserve bone density. PMDD may be driven by low levels of either progesterone or estrogen so some experimentation may be involved in discovering the appropriate level of these hormones.

Total Hysterectomy/ Oophorectomy

Small studies reported relief of PMDD when a hysterectomy and bilateral oophorectomy were performed. Hysterectomy with oophorectomy should be considered a last-resort treatment option for women with severe PMDD that has not responded to standard treatments. In a 1990 study, fourteen women with severe, debilitating PMDD volunteered for a study of therapy by hysterectomy, oophorectomy, and continuous estrogen replacement. All had completed their families and had failed to benefit from previous medical treatments. Six months after surgery, PMDD symptom charting revealed that all of the women had complete relief of symptoms. 6 months after operation, the women showed dramatic improvement in mood, general affect, well-being, life satisfaction, and overall quality of life. This study showed that surgical therapy, involving oophorectomy, hysterectomy, and continuous estrogen replacement, is effective in relieving the symptoms of PMDD.

The trouble is many of these choices involve complications of their own (for example, hysterectomy necessitates estrogen replacement, or SSRIs often have side effects) and for many women what will help is not one treatment or another, but figuring out a combination of the above.

I put out an invitation for others to share their stories of treatment options for coping with PMDD, and am thrilled to have these to share with you now:

Heidi: I was first diagnosed around 2009. I feel like I've had it for much longer, but it definitely got worse after having my children. I have always hated the idea of being on meds and always felt that I was strong enough to handle PMDD on my own. Finally around 2010 I realized that I had to do something and made the call to my doctor. She prescribed me Celexa and it honestly turned my life around. In the beginning I had to take it daily; 10mg during my normal days then increasing to 20mg then up to 30mg the worse things got. Now I'm able to just take it during my PMDD time. I start at ovulation then stop two days after I start my period. I was VERY lucky to find something that worked for me so quickly. I have to take my med at night because it makes my drowsy, but that helps with the insomnia.

Tina: I have been on and off different SSRI's for many years. Some seemed to work better than others. Presently I have been taking Lexapro 20 mg and a mood stabilizer Lamictal 100 mg for about 2 years now and they are working. I have a history of some minor depression as a result of a dysfunctional upbringing with a drinking father. I have never been diagnosed with PMDD except by myself. I figured it out about a 18 months ago after I believe suffering with it for years, possibly since I was 16 yrs old and I'm now 49. There were some things that complicated my story which made it difficult to understand what was happening to me. I had drinking issues for years and I was in a bad marriage for 16 years as well. Since I left my husband last June, although my PMDD still rears its ugly head, the symptoms have greatly improved. For one I am taking meds regularly, and I also don't have the husband blaming me and making me feel crazier.

Josephine: I just started a group of supplements on Sunday morning. I went from hysterical on Saturday and to somehow not having cried or become a psychotic bitch like I usually do. I now take multi vitamins, magnesium, Calcium, 5-htp, evening primrose oil, and flax seed. I take one of everything in the morning with a whole glass of orange juice, then take the second 5-htp and primrose with lunch. I still feel like I'm running at a higher stress level than usual but compared to my usual PMDD I feel amazing. I also just started taking a calcium, magnesium and zinc supplement. This past cycle was so much better.

Olivia: I was 16 when my PMDD symptoms started. I was on birth control and continued until I was 24. It did not help me with the symptoms of anxiety, depression, body pains, cramps or rage. When I was 17 years old I was diagnosed and treated for depression. I was put on Zoloft and saw a psychiatrist . At 19, I switch to Prozac and continued until I was 21. When I was 21 I saw a different psychiatrist who took me off of Prozac because it didn't make me feel good. I work with the psychiatrist for 10 years with just psychotherapy.

Finally, in 2013 I told my OB about my symptoms and asked her if I could by chance have a hormone imbalance? She diagnosed me with PMDD. I was happy to know. I thought "all these years thinking it was just me." She gave me Estrium made by Metagenics to take which are everyday vitamins to help with PMS symptoms and Chasteberry during PMDD Days. I teach yoga, so I found poses to be help me during those specific times, I go to Barre Method classes two times a week at least, I use breathing techniques, and my husband and I both track my PMDD time and I tell him how he can help me. I use meditation and lavender oil in a diffusor by my bed during those nights. I do a lot of steps (sometimes even when I do not feel like it) to make this work for me.

Samantha: 20mg of daily fluoxetine has been the best treatment for me by far. Birth control pills made me worse and I've recently tried

medical cannabis in lieu of Xanax for panic
attacks.

See that last one there about cannabis? I did some extra
poking around on the subject of using marijuana/THC as
a treatment option and it seems that as more states than
ever are legalizing this drug more women than ever are
giving it a go.

"I like the Zoot Drops," a woman who asked to remain
anonymous told me via email, referring to the small
bottle of blends that deliver 10mg of THC per serving. "I
find it easier to use than SSRIs because when I'm
feeling the worst it works almost immediately to chill me
out, and when I'm fine I don't need to take it at all."

She continued, "It makes me feel a little more relaxed
and a little bit numb, which isn't something I'd advocate
for on a daily basis but on the days I'm just trying to get
through to when I'm 'normal' again that bit of help is a
lifesaver. Unlike alcohol I don't end up hungover, and in
fact feel like I sleep better than my usual PMDD nights.

"I don't know if it's for everyone, but it feels right for me
right now. I'd rather take THC (without even having to
smoke it) than anything else."

Others, however, have mentioned the use of medical
marijuana gives them no relief and increases their
trouble with anxiety attacks.

Five — Reaching Out

In researching for this book I've seen other women share in private groups about their hard days in posts and pictures that hurt with their familiarity. I've seen tear-stained cheeks, read countless stories of fear and frustration, and seen undeniable evidence of self-harm. These are our friends, our mothers and sisters, hurting so deeply, and yet very little is being said about it — or even worse, when we do ask for support our truth is being downplayed.

Aside from my husband the first person I tried to confide in, even before visiting the doctor, was an old friend whom I hadn't seen in a couple of months. In the time since our last chat life had been busy for both of us. Since she was going to be moving soon as well I felt that I couldn't cancel our last lunch date even though I woke up feeling absolutely terrible. Over sandwiches and coffee I struggled to take part in the conversation, and eventually a few tears escaped. I was so embarrassed to be crying in the middle of a restaurant, but I managed to work out the words to explain I thought I had PMDD.

My friend, whom I love dearly, paused for a moment after I explained some of the feelings I had been having, and then said that sometimes she feels bad too. My hopes rose for a small second, thinking perhaps we had this in common, but then she went on to talk about how she doesn't think all days are meant to be your best and some dips are to be expected.

The advice she gave wasn't half bad but it hurt tremendously all the same. It had been so hard for me to open up and tell her how much I was suffering, and it felt like she either didn't get it or didn't believe me. To be fair, I might not have done a very good job of explaining what was going on and the severity of what I felt, but it seemed like she wanted to make it out to be just a bad day, a small divot in an otherwise good life. Honestly though, I was crying for help, waving an arm up to signal I needed to be rescued from the cycle I was drowning in. I didn't follow through with the conversation any further right then, and much to my dismay she never followed up in the weeks or months following to ask how I was doing.

My other experience sharing such personal details of my struggles came with another close friend after I'd sought help from the doctors. By then PMDD wasn't as big and scary to me as it had once been. I had wrapped my mind around the truth that this was something that was happening to me, not something that was my fault, and so when she mentioned that she thought she was going crazy I was able to lend an ear while sharing what I had been through. All in all it was a much better experience, and while I don't think there's only one right way to respond to someone who opens up to you I do believe it's important to always believe whatever they are saying.

A look at what online friends of mine had to say about reactions they've received from those they've confided in, and how they wish it had gone instead:

> Melissa: Most have no idea what it is. Others will say...my period is bad too.

Heather: When I tell people they have no idea. When I explain, they say, "Oh PMS." It is frustrating because there are times I feel PMDD debilitates me, and if others really understood they could not get upset at me. When they do not understand, and get upset, it makes it even more depressing.

Joy: The best thing to say to someone who has PMDD is something that lets them know you understand they do not choose to be that way and you know it isn't just an excuse. That you hope it improves.

Stephanie: People have said: PM...what? What is that? You have that? So you get really bad periods? Everyone gets crazy on their periods! Best thing to say to someone with PMDD: I am here if you need me. Don't be afraid to let me know if you need or want me for anything, ok?

Jen: Sometimes if PMDD is ruining my day/life, rather than try to explain it to someone, I lie. There are days I CAN'T get out of bed. There is no way to explain it to someone who doesn't have PMDD, because they don't understand, and don't get it. They think things about me as a person that are not true. Then it becomes a confrontation that exasperates the issues even more. It pains me to have to lie. I have a guilty conscience sometimes. But, there isn't a way to convince ignorant people that it is a real problem. It is horrible and has ruined a lot of things for me.

Piper: Can you imagine if I called into work for my PMDD? The other 24 women I work with would be like "I PMS too and I still work..what is her problem...suck it up." So instead I get a migraines or have the flu.

Claire: I miss church at times, and appointments and different events. I will not even attempt to tell people why, because they just look at me with a blank stare and think I'm being ridiculous. It hurts.

Beth: People truly have no idea what is really going on, what the days are actually like. I get the feeling people think it is an excuse or that I am weak by the way they react. They do not realize how much intense effort it takes just to get through the day, often hiding everything. I have been called selfish because of canceling plans and/or not following through with things. To me, the best things people can do are the small things likes texts or messages that remind me I'm not the horrible monster that I feel like. Small, thoughtful words. And be there when it's over! It's nice to be together with people after and know that they still love you. That's important to me, to know that when I'm back to myself people still want to be with me and haven't given up. This is what will keep me going through the next one, knowing people will still be there.

Amy: I used to say it's really bad PMS. I felt I wasn't taken seriously, and I was an exaggerator. I now can explain it as "it's a mood disorder caused by my hormones not mixing with my brain chemistry. It's a medical problem." I typically don't tell anyone. Very few know that I have it, other than close family, I sometimes have sent them pics from these FB groups. I don't feel the need to tell people because no one knows what it is, including doctors.

Maria: I've been told that many times by my husband that I use it as an excuse to use him as my pin cushion. I have said I don't want to act like this. He also told me if I know it's PMDD I should be able to control what I say. I said it doesn't work that way. I don't care during PMDD because I'm raging.

To anyone who might be wondering what a good way to respond to such a reveal is I'd advise making listening and believing your top priorities. If someone says they are hurting they mean it. Thank them for trusting you enough to be someone they can confide in, and ask if there's anything you can do to help. Most likely the answer will be no, but the offer is invaluable.

Six — Is PMDD Real?

Complicating everything, the questions of if PMDD is real and if women's emotions need to be medicated at all continues to be asked.

From a post titled "Is PMDD Real?" published in 2002 by American Psychological Association:

> "It's a real biological condition for which women seek treatment--and for which effective treatment is available," says Jean Endicott, PhD, director of the premenstrual evaluation unit at Columbia Presbyterian Medical Center.
>
> Eight years ago it was included in the Diagnostic and Statistical Manual of Mental Disorders, Fourth Edition (DSM-IV). But many health professionals say PMDD does not exist, that it can be confused with other mental health disorders, such as depression. Psychologists in this camp contend women shouldn't have to be diagnosed with a mental illness in order for others to believe they are uncomfortable or unhappy or to get help and support.
>
> Referencing Paula Caplan, PhD, who is the author of "They Say You're Crazy" the article goes on to explain:
>
> Some feminist psychologists like Caplan believe that the language surrounding PMDD is misleading and that its classification as a

psychiatric disorder stigmatizes women as mentally ill and covers up the real reasons of women's anguish. "It's a label that can be used by a sexist society that wants to believe that many women go crazy once a month," Caplan explains.

"Women are supposed to be cheerleaders," she adds. "When a woman is anything but that, she and her family are quick to think something is wrong."

Meanwhile, for women, the controversy can be frustrating and confusing. Those who experience severe premenstrual changes just want some relief.

Can I get an 'amen' on that last note? All I know is it sure as shit feels real, and as I recently told an online friend, "If this is normal for a woman then I don't want to be it."

I feel abnormal, and though I get the other side of the argument (in an online discussion just yesterday a woman explained how she feels her emotions are running out of control and a man replied: "And women wonder why they'll never really be equal." Ugh.) I also feel compelled to be honest about myself and my struggles.

Caplan went on to write in a 2008 article for feminist.org:

Frantic to be loving, nurturant and serene, women learn to pathologize themselves, often ignoring the real causes of their upset. It seems less daunting to say, "It must be hormonal!" than to begin the frightening process of looking at underlying causes and realizing, for instance, "I need to leave this job—or relationship." Many have claimed the PMDD label for themselves and asked for medication, hoping for a quick solution.

I don't even know what else to say other than that I've had PMS, wanted to slap it across its face and challenge it to a carbohydrate-eating competition, but then was ready to move on. PMS is annoying, PMDD is debilitating.

What Caplan is saying feels so much like downplaying my cry for help it angers me. It just does not make sense that 2 to 3 weeks of the month I have a happy home and work life and the remainder of the time I'm a complete wreck because I'd rather think of myself as too much of a weak, hormonal person than to address the "real causes" of my upset.

I have no real qualifications with which to argue against Caplan and others who claim it's not in the best interest of women to see PMDD medications and cures researched other than my own personal experience and the ears with which I've listened to hundreds of women out there like myself.

Aside from addressing their points with my own experiences the truth is I feel daunted by trying to figure out what PMDD means on the grand scale during my low days, and too busy on my good days to try and figure out. (You know, being "frantic" about being seen as nurturing and serene /sarcasm.) It feels like a conversation too big for me right now, and all I truly care about is making sure those that feel they are in need of help know how to get it and feel no shame in doing so.

My plate is full, my person is tired. This is a battle I choose not to fight right now.

Seven — Those Who Live With Us Living With PMDD

Because I've written before about PMDD I occasionally get messages from women who suspect they have it, or those who love them. Through Facebook I received this message from a man (whose name and any identifying details have been changed) asking for help with his wife:

Hi, saw your post about PMDD. I am worried sick that my marriage may crumble because my wife has it and it remains unaddressed. If I bring it up I'm the sexist pig who thinks her fears, concerns worries, are all part of her womanly curse. And so there I stand, enduring an enormous screaming dress down for leaving the vacuum cleaner where it doesn't belong, being called names in front of my kids that I wouldn't use on a malicious stranger. I look in the waste basket upstairs and know that this is her time. In 5-6 days, she will be my amazing, hardworking, loving, happy wife again. What do I do? Is there any way to broach this subject with her?

I felt honored that he had reached out to me, and did my best to reply with what I thought was practical advice:

Hey there, thanks for reaching out and sorry to hear about what you've been going through.

I'm absolutely no expert on this, and know only what I've experienced firsthand. That being said, I would try and broach the subject a week or so after you believe she's had her period. At that time she ought to be the most level-headed and hopefully more open to hearing you than just reacting emotionally.

As for how to do it, well, that's tricky but one way to do it might be to start by telling her you've had some concerns for a while now and did a bit of Googling. Maybe show her the post(s) I wrote and ask her to read them. Then try and find out if she feels like any of it rings true to her.

Hopefully that will get some talk going, but at the very least I'd stand up for yourself and say it's unacceptable to have yelling and name-calling in front of the kids. If she doesn't agree on that point, well, that's a red flag of other huge issues. Assuming she does agree, try and think up a way together to tell the other person when they're entering dangerous territory.

This is totally stupid, but totally works for my husband and me.

A year or so ago I got totally fed up with his little jokes going on and on, and him not being able to tell when I'd truly had enough (my tolerance varies greatly depending on my mood). One day I said to him, "See how I'm waving my arm like this [motion like you'd do sticking your arm out a car window to feel the breeze] that's our new secret signal that you're irritating the shit out of me and you need to stop or I'm going to get genuinely mad." When I do it now we both laughed because it's just damn ridiculous looking.

Not only has it worked as a way for us to understand immediately what I'm saying without having to even use words, but he'll use it on me too when I'm pestering about this or that and not getting his hints to just let it go. Perhaps if you two established something like this she could be more clear about when she's at a tipping point and you could also have a word-free way to tell her she's going too far.

While it's hard that there doesn't seem to be any easy solutions to PMDD, I'll leave you with hope. Just as it seemed to start for me over a couple of months when I'd never had it for years and years before, it does seem to be dissipating. Everyone is different, but keep in mind there's a possibility you both won't always be having to deal with this.

Did that sounds suspiciously upbeat to you? In hindsight, replying during one of my normal times may not have been the best idea. Four days after feeling like I had a handle on PMDD, just when I could almost glimpse it in my rearview mirror, I spent entire day in bed tearing up over Project Runway reruns (those designers' dreams being dashed!). I don't even like reality television.

Remember that list of symptoms from way in the beginning? The one that hurts me the most is "lasting irritability or anger that affects other people." Ugh. It's like a knife to the heart that amplifies the guilt factor as it slides so easily through. I find it tremendously hard to deal with myself when I'm having PMDD, and having to deal with those dealing with me is a whole other mess. I feel for the man who sent me that email, as well as his wife.

My kids, the ones who I'm ashamed to have screamed at, know at this point that sometimes their mama doesn't feel good. They must have noticed by now I go to bed before them far more often than their father, and surely feel that sometimes they don't know what they're going to get when they interact with me.

Heartache, I know thee.

Thus far I've kept the explanations to them incredibly simple. "I'm not feeling very good today," I'll say as I bow out early in the evening to hide in bed. If they see me crying I try to be at least partially honest and say something like, "I'm feeling upset today. There isn't anything you need to worry about, though. I think if I get a good night's sleep I'll feel much better in the morning."

As they age I plan to more forthright about what's really going on, piggybacking off the sex education they'll get at school. "You know how you learned today that girls have their period every month?" I imagine I'll say. "Well, sometimes when that happens they feel moody, like angry or frustrated or sad. That's what happens to me. It's not easy to deal with, but I know I can get through it and after a couple of days of feeling bad I start to feel better."

Parenting hasn't come particularly easy to me and so I won't even bother to pretend I know for sure this is the best approach, but I've always been age-appropriately honest with my children. On top of offering information at a rate I feel they're ready for I have an open-door policy on questions. They can ask me anything and I'll answer with the truth. If it somehow turns out they want to know more about my mood swings or how female bodies work I'll tell them, in as much detail as they want, and perhaps someday way down the line they'll even read this book.

As far as the husband goes, I'm incredibly blessed to have a good 'picker.' Boy howdy, I'm lucky that the man I fell in love with is incredibly patient and understanding — even though there was a learning curve to this whole PMDD thing that was bumpy as hell.

The first time I "quit" life and shut myself in the bedroom for the day he was pissed. I did not, at that time, recognize or have the words to communicate what I was going through, and I believe he thought I was completely ridiculous. A mom of two refusing to come out of her room when her in-laws are over? Who does that?! His reaction hurt me even further, but I can't say it wasn't understandable. I didn't know what was going on, couldn't explain it, and was an absolutely mysterious mess.

Over time, as I learned about PMDD and recognized myself in the list of symptoms, I shared everything with him from the Wikipedia basics to posts by other women in Facebook groups. "Doesn't this sound so much like me?" I'd ask excitedly, forcing him to read about the troubles another woman was going through. "I think I've said those exact same words before!"

Together we learned, but to be perfectly honest he was a better student than I. He got it, almost immediately, and began to act as my sounding board.

"I almost wish I could videotape you," he said to me, as I blubbered away one month about my frustrations and feelings of failure. "If I showed you this next week you'd laugh at how obvious it is you're feeling low right now."

Oddly enough, he was so right that I did laugh right then and there. Being able to tell someone I trust completely things like, "If how I feel right now is who I really am then I am a miserable, terrible human being," and have them know how to handle it is the best. We wade our way through the low times together, me using my best "I feel…" statements in high frequency, and him doling out reality checks on an as-needed basis.

There is one kind of conversation he refuses to have, however. Any sentence I begin with "What if…" immediately gets a laugh and a dismissive shake of the head. In the early months we went down the road paved by anxiety and had endless, circling conversations about all the things in the future that could possibly go wrong: the Bird Flu, a car accident, cancer, juvenile delinquents, runaways, house fires, kidnappers, drug addiction, mental illness, poverty. The list went on, and on, and on, and once the jar of worms had been opened no answer he could give could satisfy my ramped up brain — and so we stopped. "What if" conversations are no longer indulged in, and we're both better for it.

It's a bit of a surprise to me that I'm a proponent of burying your fears and seeking distraction (hello Netflix binge-watching), but the years I've been dealing with PMDD-induced anxiety have taught me there isn't really anything to be gained by going there. If anything, it's damaging to allow myself step off that cliff (whether with a co-conversationist or by myself), and so House of Cards it is. If that thing that I am so very worried about at that moment is truly that important I will be able to mull it over in a week when I have two steady feet are under me.

In order to make sure I'm ready to dole out the "I feel…" statements before it's too late I use a period tracking app. Right now I'm working with the free app Period Diary, which is filled with I-don't-quite-get-the-correlation flowers, but handy all the same.

Here's a look at what my fellow PMDD survivors had to say when I asked how their families cope with their low times:

> Gail: I have a very supportive husband. We've just recently started to openly discuss PMDD and those times of the month when I seem to be going crazy. He's very patient with me and he thinks twice before saying anything that might upset me. He's willing and able to take over the household if I need to rest or just hide away for awhile. It wasn't always this easy though. We've been into some near wars in my house. With knowing the symptoms of PMDD I'm not longer scared to share all of my thoughts with him and to get them out of my head is so relieving.

> Sophia: As far as my 8 yr old daughter. I am really just beginning to have talks with her regarding what's going on with me. In my opinion, she is at a perfect age to really begin to understand this.

> Beth: I tell my kids the truth, very open with them when I change meds or when I am getting frustrated or upset about things or why I am sad.. ect. My kids are 9,13 and 15 and I have been open with them for a few years now. I feel it's better for them to know then to be confused

as to why their mom always seen like someone else.

Kris: I recently shared what I go through with my own mom and she said that she thinks she had PMDD before she had her hysterectomy. It's probably best that I share with my daughter about what's going on if she is destined to deal with it too.

Aimee: I've never had anyone stick around (relationship wise)- I push them away, or they just can't handle the baggage. I am very straight with everyone, family, children, friends- of what I go through and what is happening with me. My children are very supportive and understanding. They know my 'crazy time' and about cycles. We have our coping strategies as well as supportive friends.

Janelle: I told my kids that with my period comes hormonal changes that cause me to get very irritable and that when I'm like that I want them to know how I love them even when I am grouchy. I do my best to trudge through the horrible feelings I have and to continue to show them love anyway. Not easy but its getting better. I wish my ex-husband to be would have helped by being emotionally there for me but he was not. He blamed me for everything..even his own bad moods.

Marcy: Make sure they have an outlet. Writing, dancing, even just a quiet zone to chill out in when moms grouchy... When I'm feeling overwhelmed by sounds, the kids go to their rec room and color or play with Lego (on the carpet because I can't stand the sound of Lego lol)- I made sure they have a playroom that's Bitchy Mom proof. There's room for my dancing daughter, zone for the gamers, books, movies, craft stuff... It's a haven actually when they need to space themselves.

Lena: My family has been extremely supportive and I've been honest about what hormones are and why when they are out if whack it makes us feel ill and moody. My 8 year old son is a born nurturer and will hug me, rub my back and doesn't get distressed at my tears. My 14 yr old son son will also hug me and has shown great maturity dealing with it. I've learned to recognize when the hormones are putting me in a bad place and just tell them what my needs are and they roll with it. My husband had been my rock although when we first started going through insomnia/anxiety attacks he was frustrated: now that he knows what this is all about, he can often talk me off the ledge do to speak. Believe me, I know how blessed I am with all three!

Holly: I am very open with my son. As a single mom I don't really have the luxury of keeping it from him. Plus, it caused more problems keeping him in the dark. Now that he knows that I have a medical condition that causes mood swings, he doesn't feel like he is a bad kid or is at fault without really understanding why. I have other medical issues, so he is involved in those as well, which has helped alleviate his anxiety. My mom has been more supportive as her understanding of this disease has grown - it has been a blessing. My dad tries but doesn't really understand.

Jen: My husband and I set up a code word that he can tell me when I am not myself, because I don't realize I'm not in my right mind. My kids know that mom has "sick weeks" and I spend as much time as possible alone

Grace: The more literature I show my husband the more understanding he seems to be however our past experiences have shown a complete lack of understanding or sympathy towards what I go through. My mother and sister say they get it but make no allowances for when I lose it so I know they really don't. My boys - age 8 and 10 - just think mommy is in bed all the time - that sucks.

Eight — Getting On with It

These days I make my way not with medication, but by subsisting on coffee (hallelujah), healthy food (for the most part) and gummy vitamins (pills make me barf ever damn time). My personal door to taking drugs isn't entirely closed, and if a time comes that I feel the need to try birth control or SSRIs again I will do so without thinking twice. In the meantime, I spend my low days trying tremendously hard to cut myself some slack.

For a long time, in my tiny jacked-up brain, I was convinced I was the one to blame for this happening over and over. I thought I somehow I caused this monstrous beast to appear again and again, and if I were only a better, stronger person my whole family wouldn't have to be burdened by it. I'm wrong quite a lot, thankfully, and I was decidedly wrong on that particular note. It took me years to learn it wasn't my fault, and now I desperately want others to recognize it isn't theirs either.

When I wake up in a mood so black I question every single thing in my life and feel an itch to throw it all out the window I cross whatever exercise goal I had in mind off the to-do list and force myself to accept that lying low is a real option. If that means not leaving the house for an entire day, then so be it. If that means making pancakes, smothering them in peanut butter, drizzling them with syrup, and scarfing them down while finding out who could not outwit, outplay or outlast the others in 2002, then so be it. I grab my cats, climb into bed, and fight with all of my might not to give into the self-loathing thoughts.

I've even gotten creative and enlisted the help of my sister-in-law to tackle some of my frustrations, which I didn't even correlate were PMDD-related until I saw another sufferer comment online that she has Misophonia, which literally translates to "hatred of sound." I have sensitive ears on any given day, but when I'm feeling low they go into overdrive to the point I can actually hear the fibers of my pillow creaking as I try and fall asleep. Sounds crazy, right? I know, but between that and living with a partner who doesn't sleep very well in general and so is always using his tablet and phone I was going nutty.

Sick of the noise and lights, but uncomfortable in a traditional sleep mask with side straps, I doodled up a soft hat that has the sleep mask portion hanging off the front and she was kind enough to sew one for me. Flip it up if you need to see, down when you're in do-not-disturb mode. It's soft and cozy, does wonders for blocking things like the glare from the light on the smoke alarm and dampens sounds just a bit. Oh, the lengths we'll go to when something is annoying us to no end!

Because I'm now in the know about PMDD, and can predict when my lowest times will be, I plan ahead. I literally mark my calendars so that as I look ahead I can see when I may not be feeling up for social interactions or work commitments. I am tremendously lucky to be able to work even a little bit ahead as a freelance writer, and therefore can plan for when I need to take a break, or at the very least have a slow production day.

I wonder sometimes, how those of you out there with PMDD and real jobs manage, and then the thoughts begin need to creep in. "Not only are you weak," they say, "but you are among the weakest of them all. You can barely even handle a work-from-home job."

See how they so sneakily do their thing?

It's incredibly tempting to follow that line of thinking and place myself at the very bottom of those who suffer, as a weaker and more pathetic than all the rest, but I won't. I can't let myself. If trying to talk myself out of it doesn't quickly work then I will either turn to a support group to express what I'm feeling or find a distraction.

It's a gamble, every month, as the numbers tick down to the dark days, whether or not I'm making the right choice to go drug-free or not. I hate never knowing how long or how intense my PMDD feelings are going to be. I hate that I even have to think about it at all, and yet I feel most often this is the right path for me right now. Please know this is just my story, and you should do whatever you feel is right for you.

Perhaps I'm delusional, continually suffering from the post-period amnesia I experienced so intensely in my early PMDD days, but I do believe my symptoms are slowly getting less intense over the months and years. Not every month consistently, but overall. Even without drugs it's been months and months since I've locked myself away for an entire day.

For other women though, their PMDD days are great in number and strong in severity. Where my mood-affected days are down to a handful others are in the double-digits. Where my periods, with the cramps and bloating and uncomfortableness nearly all women know, are just a couple of days, others are a week or longer. Combine a full week of mood symptoms and a full week of menstruation together and it's overwhelming. Half of your life! That's 182.5 days a year being lost to feeling unwell. My heart and deepest sympathies go out to anyone dealing with such a high amount of life disruption.

Despite considering myself 'lucky' in having not as many days intruded upon I often feel as though I've been through the ringer. Occasionally I want to stomp my foot and protest that I've had more than my fair share of hardships, but I will say that having PMDD has also given me a great empathy for others who are dealing with mood disorders or mental illness. It scares me to admit it, but I get how easily a life can be derailed. The line between doing well and falling apart is frighteningly thin.

It's not easy to find a way to give thanks for what is arguably the hardest part of my life and others' lives, but I've seen some amazing reflection happening. Some find such low times give them extra reason to be thankful for the good times, and others hold onto in the small things their loved ones do to try and help them feel better.

A look at how friends of mine say they get through the worst of it:

> Elizabeth: I *would remind myself that what happens today, my kids remember tomorrow, or 30 years from now. Focusing on them (and the childhood memories they'd have) really helped me try to control it the best I could. I'd go to my

room for a few minutes to cool down. When I did lose my temper, I'd apologize every time after I'd cooled off. I had to remind myself it was just a time game. "Just one more week" or "just a couple more days and I'll be me again".

*I use past tense because I just had a full abdominal hysterectomy. I specifically asked for my ovaries to be removed (at 28 yo) to rid myself of this terrible disorder.

Victoria: The only way that I am able to keep moving forward is because I know that in Christ I am perfect and whole. The Bible promises that God has plans for us - for hope and a future - and when I can I focus on that. I would not be here today if it weren't for my faith in God. We do get more than we can handle in life - but God is with us and in us to help us through that which we cannot handle alone. I'm so thankful for that!

May: Chocolate in vast amounts,I clear my diary of non essentials if I'm very bad.I'm also trying cbt (cognitive behavioral therapy) and reflexology.

Sylvia: Exercise is the very best break from PMDD, that and being outside, and knowing that you will catch a break on your normal weeks.

Julia: Don't give up. Don't accept no or "I don't know" as answers. Be your own advocate. Be open with your kids, they are more understanding & forgiving than adults if you are honest with them. Give yourself a break - some things won't matter in a few years so let those things go. Prioritize - put the truly important things first. Do what you need to & don't let others bully/persuade/convince you to do something you don't want to.

Gwen: All I can say , BRAINPOWER & trying to always keep faith & never lose hope. Brain power is big for me. I'm forever fighting my own destructive thinking. I'm very stubborn & assertive by nature so therefore I WILL NOT let this win!!! I fall down ALOT but keep finding the STRENGTH to get back up.

Nine — Going Public with PMDD

The full truth is I've had a very hard time deciding
whether or not I should put my real name on the cover of
this very book. I've wrestled with the decision while
feeling at my worst, tears pouring out from frustration
over my inability to decide. I've also put off the decision
until I was feeling better and was still unable to decide.

It's daunting to consider telling everyone you know and a
whole host of strangers the very worst parts about
yourself. Do I forever want the Googling of my name to
turn up results about someone who outright admits their
frame of mind is at times untrustworthy? If I were to ever
go and get a 'real' job (not that being a writer isn't one,
but it's a different kind of job, certainly) what will my
potential employer think? Will this book keep me from
being hired?

These are obvious questions, I feel, but on an even
more personal level I worry what will change with those I
see face-to-face. Not with my husband, who has long
heard all about how I'm feeling in extensive detail, but
with those I wasn't brave enough or ready enough to
share it with. Will my parents be hurt I didn't share with
them I was feeling so low? Will our acquaintances think
differently of me? Will their heads tilt just the tiniest bit
out of concern when they ask how I've been?

These questions are enough to make my stomach
churn, but they're not just mine. They're yours too. Have

you been open in talking about your struggles? Why or why not?

Finally, over three months of considering the questions in my sound mind and with emotions taking the wheel, I realized something I recognized a while ago — it's not my fault. I am not weak for having PMDD, just as someone who has been diagnosed with cancer did not get it because they are weak. Shit happens. You get an unlucky roll of the dice, a bad hand or some other gambling/life analogy, and then the lot is yours to deal with. I may not be proud at this moment of having PMDD, but it's also nothing I should be ashamed about.

I had to ask myself, if I hide behind a pen name what does that mean? On the plus side it would mean privacy, but other than that not much. Conversely, not using my own name would demonstrate shame, which weighs on me infinitely. It would mean telling my story but not being brave enough to own it, and I fear that would have left me in a much worse state than worrying about some possible-but-probably-not-going-to-even-happen employer or ex-boyfriend Googling me up and finding out I'm a real human, faults and all.

Coincidentally, I saw a post from Glennon Doyle Melton of Momastery recently, in which she wrestled with whether or not to reveal her struggles with bulimia to a group of people in the Dominican Republic. The tears spilled over as I read her recollection of the speech she was pushed into giving:

> "[The audience] looked at each other and shifted in their chairs and then they seemed to collectively sit up straighter. I panicked again.

Did they understand bulimia? Would I have to explain it? How the hell would I explain that I had so much food that I ate and ate and threw it up in the toilet and ate some more to people without enough food? I thought about being really, really ashamed of my horrible, ridiculous, wasteful, American, self-harming self. But then I told myself: STOP IT. NO. Glennon—refuse to be ashamed of your problems and they'll not be ashamed of theirs. That's how it works. At home and everywhere else, probably. CARRY ON. I carried on."

Glennon's post led me to the TedTalks of Dr. Brené Brown and like magic the words I needed poured out of the computer directly at me. Never mind that her two presentations were given in 2010 and 2012, these word were meant for exactly for me on that very day in 2015.

You see, I have felt shame about having PMDD but I'm working on stepping out of it. Even just announcing to friends, family and a few strangers that I had this book in the works left me with an "shame hangover" (as Brené calls it) the next day, during which I didn't even leave the house. I've been too scared to tell most people in my real life that I have really hard days and I have no idea what the hell I'm doing attempting to tell so many others. I feel simultaneously like doing this hard thing is the very right thing to do and utterly vulnerable in doing it.

In the many years I've been writing I've seen all kind of comments come in on the blogs and know for certain there are trolls out there waiting to strike. I got used to it though, when writing about the celebrities or latest parenting fad, because there was a wall of topic between us. If I really write about my real self (and I'm even considering sharing some photos) I'm terrified the bad comments will come and they'll hit hard. I don't know if I can take it with no buffer.

Somehow I talked myself into this still, but then the pendulum swung a different way. "Who are you to think you ought to write an entire book about yourself?" the thoughts jabbed. "You're not good enough to be who everyone is going to think you're trying to be — a leader of a cause — and they know it."

Enter again Brené Brown. In the second of her TEDTalks she says:

> "Shame drives two big tapes -- 'never good enough' and, if you can talk it out of that one, 'who do you think you are?' The thing to understand about shame is it's not guilt. Shame is a focus on self, guilt is a focus on behavior. Shame is 'I am bad.' Guilt is 'I did something bad.'"

"I am bad?"

Is that something I believe to be true? I actually think not. PMDD is bad, not I am bad. Maybe I'm not ashamed.

That thought felt like a lightbulb moment.

I'm not usually one for self-help category, but today I'm gathering up my Glennon bravery and my Brené smarts, as well as my Oprah enthusiasm and Stuart Smalley assurances. I'm stepping out into the public with this, because this is the full me. PMDD sucks, but it's not my fault, and I want anyone else out there living with it to know it isn't there's either.

The evening after the coffee spilling incident I cooked all the vegetables in the house because I tend to go into overdrive about the way we eat when I've got guilt going on over not being how I'd like to be. Spaghetti squash, zucchini, red pepper, cauliflower, Brussels sprouts and even leeks (how does one even properly cook such a thing?) sizzled away as I thought about our rough start to the day — and then the smoke alarm went off.

My two boys jumped into action (sadly, this is far from the first time this has happened, but I swear it's over active alarms rather than THAT bad of cooking to blame), grabbing towels and whirling them over their heads to clear the air and make the ear-piercing beeping stop.

"Thank you," I said to them when it finally ceased. "I appreciate you helping without even being asked to so much."

Three minutes later the buggers assaulted us with their noise again.

Boys jumped up with grins on their faces and went back into whirling action, and I grinned right along. By then the morning coffee had been made and spilled, made again and drank. I'd committed a motherhood sin by shouting at my children, and they'd forgiven. With the breeze from the towels in the air I got a small hint of a sense that we'll make it through. It's going to be messy, for sure, but we'll make it.

Ultimately, I think the number one thing that has helped me deal with living with PMDD is realizing that there's no one at fault here to be blamed and shamed, which is the very reason for the title of this book — we need to talk about PMDD. In researching more about this subject I have seen woman after woman express relief upon finding a Facebook group or message board where information and support are available. Most of them have only recently heard of the condition, are so thankful to find out they're not actually going crazy, and are tremendously grateful not to be alone.

Conversely, not knowing what's going on combined with feelings of self loathing, insufficiency, despair and anxiety is a dangerous combination. Our friends, our sisters, our women are suffering and many of them are under the delusion their families and loved ones would be better off without them. Suicidal ideation (also known as suicidal thoughts about how to kill oneself, which can range from a detailed plan to a fleeting consideration) are had by many going through PMDD. That's scary as hell, and we need to reach anyone feeling that way.

If you do happen to be a reality television watcher you may remember Gia Allemand, who appeared on both The Bachelor and Bachelor Pad. The beauty, who also was featured in Maxim, died at the young age of 29. On August 12, 2013, she was admitted to University Hospital in New Orleans after an attempted suicide by hanging. She was declared brain dead and removed from life support two days later.

I'm 33 as the writing of this book, and that gives me chills.

Donna, who is the late star's mother, described being on the phone with her daughter when she attempted suicide while speaking to Dr. Phil:

> "At that point, with how she felt with her menstrual cycle, she could not see clearly ... It was like night and day. It would come out of nowhere. All of a sudden, something would click in there and she would say 'This isn't right. He doesn't love me.'"

Donna went on to share Gia had been upset about recent fights with her boyfriend, NBA star Ryan Anderson, and another family member but believes the hormonal extremes are what pushed her daughter over the edge. It's a statement Dr. Christina Charbonneau, who wrote an article for SheKnows about Gia's death and PMDD, appears to concur with.

Sports Illustrated wrote about Ryan trying to recover from Gia's suicide in late 2014:

> Ryan's first response was to shut down. He moved back in with his parents and ate only when his mother forced him to, and even then just applesauce and yogurt. His sister, Rachel, and her husband, Mark Groves, took turns sleeping next to him in his queen bed. Ryan spent his days on the patio, in the baking heat, reading his Bible in silence. He couldn't bring himself to talk to his best friends, terrified of

someone saying, 'I'm sorry.' Of someone wanting him to talk about what happened."

I hate to even say it, but I fear Ryan and his family may not be the only ones trying to or who will have to recover from such a loss. Please join me in talking about PMDD with others in whatever way you are able to. You never know who you'll reach.

For suicide prevention help please click here. You can also call the National Suicide Prevention Lifeline any time at 1-800-273-8255.

Over the course of writing this book I've worked with the fine people at National Association for Premenstrual Dysphoric Disorder. My intentions here are easily summed up in this sentence of their mission statement:

> Our goal is to connect with as many women as possible that may currently have PMDD or suspect that they might, guide them to proper care, and provide them with the tools they need to reduce interpersonal conflicts and self-harm.

It's fantastic, and I highly suspect the best way to reach as many women as possible is to revamp the way we show ourselves.

I wonder, what would happen if instead of carefully cropping photos of ourselves so that our houses look cleaner and our smiles brighter we shared the real thing? What would happen if we told the truth in our status updates about how we feel rather than going silent on the bad days? Will we be attacked and accused of being attention mongers, or will we be praised for showing honesty? Will we reach someone else out there who's hurting and alone? I'm both scared and eager to find out.

I'm going to work on being more open about my mood changes by taking one picture a day that sums up how I'm feeling. You're invited to follow along and participate by connecting with my Instagram account (instagram.com/ksarasarah/), as well as to connect with me on Twitter (@Sara_McGinnis) and Facebook (facebook.com/saramcginnisonline).

Sara McGinnis' debut novel, about a woman in over her head, will be released in Summer 2015. To connect and receive updates please visit SaraMcGinnis.com and submit your email address.

Made in the USA
San Bernardino, CA
04 November 2015